HEARTBURN AND ACID REFLUX

Things you should know about heartburn and acid reflux

Dr Rowan Theo

CHAPTER ONE

Ways to Prevent Heartburn and Acid Reflux

Most folks are all too acquainted with the painful, burning sensation in the middle of the chest that's related to heartburn.

In fact, as much as 28% of adults in North America revel in gastroesophageal reflux disease (GERD), a common circumstance that reasons heartburn. GERD happens whilst acid is driven up from the belly again into the esophagus, which results in the heartburn sensation.

Although humans regularly use medicines to deal with acid reflux disease disorder and heartburn, many life-style adjustments also can assist you lessen signs and enhance your exceptional of life.

Here are 14 herbal methods to lessen your acid reflux disease disorder and heartburn, all sponsored with the aid of using clinical studies.

five Home Remedies for Heartburn and Acid Reflux

minute, four seconds

1. Chew gum

A few older research have proven that chewing gum may also assist lower acidity in the esophagus

Gum that includes bicarbonate seems to be specially powerful, as it could assist neutralize acid to save you reflux.

Chewing gum also can growth saliva production, which may also assist clean the esophagus of acid.

However, extra updated studies is wanted to decide whether or not chewing gum can assist deal with acid reflux disease disorder or relieve the signs of heartburn.

SUMMARY

Chewing gum will increase the formation of saliva and can assist clean the esophagus of belly acid.

2. Sleep to your left facet

Several research have observed that snoozing to your proper facet may also get worse reflux signs at night time .

In fact, in line with one overview, mendacity to your left facet may also lower acid publicity in the esophagus with the aid of using as much as 71%.

Although the motive isn't totally clean, it may be defined with the aid of using anatomy.

The esophagus enters the proper facet of the belly. As a result, the decrease esophageal sphincter sits above the extent of belly acid whilst you sleep to your left facet.

On the opposite hand, whilst you lie to your proper facet, belly acid covers the decrease esophageal sphincter, growing the chance of reflux .

While snoozing at the left facet all night time might not usually be possible, it may assist make you extra cushty as you fall asleep.

SUMMARY

If you revel in acid reflux disease disorder at night time, attempt snoozing at the left facet of your frame.

3 Elevate the pinnacle of your mattress

Some humans revel in reflux signs in the course of the night time, that may have an effect on sleep exceptional and make it extra hard to fall asleep .

Changing the placement which you sleep in with the aid of using raising the pinnacle of your mattress ought to assist lessen signs of acid reflux disease disorder and enhance sleep exceptional.

One overview of 4 research observed that raising the pinnacle of the mattress reduced acid reflux disease disorder and stepped forward signs like heartburn and regurgitation in humans with

Another take a look at confirmed that folks that used a wedge to raise their higher frame at the same time as snoozing skilled much less acid reflux disease disorder in comparison with once they slept flat .

SUMMARY

Elevating the pinnacle of your mattress may also lessen your reflux signs at night time.

CHAPTER TWO

Eat dinner in advance

Healthcare experts regularly endorse humans with acid reflux disease disorder to keep away from ingesting in the three hours earlier than they visit sleep.

That's due to the fact mendacity horizontally after a meal makes digestion extra hard, probably worsening GERD signs.

ingesting a past due-dinner party elevated acid publicity whilst mendacity down with the aid of using five%, in comparison with ingesting in advance in the nighttime.

Another take a look at together with humans with kind 2 diabetes observed that ingesting dinner past due at night time become related to a better chance of acid reflux disease disorder.

Still, extra research are wished earlier than strong conclusions may be made approximately the impact of past due nighttime food on GERD. It might also rely on the individual.

SUMMARY

Observational research advise that ingesting near bedtime may also get worse acid reflux disease disorder signs at night time.

However, the proof is inconclusive, and extra research are wished.

5 Opt for cooked onions in place of uncooked

Raw onions are a common cause for acid reflux disease disorder and heartburn.

One older take a look at in humans with acid reflux disease disorder confirmed that ingesting a meal containing uncooked onion notably elevated heartburn, acid reflux disease disorder, and burping, in comparison with ingesting an same meal that didn't comprise onions.

More common burping may advise that extra fueloline is being produced. This will be because of the excessive quantities of fermentable fiber in onions.

Raw onions also are extra hard to digest and may worsen the liner of the esophagus, inflicting worsened heartburn.

Whatever the motive, in case you suppose ingesting uncooked onion makes your signs worse, you have to keep away from it and choose cooked onions instead.

SUMMARY

Some humans revel in worsened heartburn and different reflux signs after ingesting uncooked onions.

6. Eat smaller, extra common food

There's a ring-like muscle referred to as the decrease esophageal sphincter in which the esophagus opens into the belly.

It acts as a valve and commonly prevents the acidic contents of the belly from going up into the esophagus. It normally remains closed however may also open whilst you swallow, belch, or vomit.

In humans with acid reflux disease disorder, this muscle is weakened or dysfunctional. Acid reflux also can arise whilst there's an excessive amount of strain at the muscle, inflicting acid to squeeze via the opening.

Unsurprisingly, maximum reflux signs take location after a meal. It additionally appears that ingesting simply one to 2 big food according to day may also get worse reflux signs.

Therefore, ingesting smaller, extra common food during the day may also assist lessen signs of acid reflux disease disorder.

SUMMARY

Acid reflux generally will increase after food, and large food appear to make it worse. Therefore, ingesting smaller, extra common food can be beneficial.

CHAPTER THREE

Maintain a mild weight

The diaphragm is a muscle positioned above your belly. Normally, the diaphragm clearly strengthens the decrease esophageal sphincter, which prevents immoderate quantities of belly acid from leaking up into the esophagus.

However, when you have extra stomach fats, the strain on your stomach may also end up so excessive that the decrease esophageal sphincter receives driven upward, far from the diaphragm's support.

Achieving and preserving a mild frame weight can assist lessen acid reflux disease disorder in the lengthy term.

However, in case you're interested by this approach, ensure to talk with a healthcare expert to evaluate whether or not it's proper for you, and if so, how you may shed pounds properly and sustainably.

SUMMARY

Losing stomach fats and preserving a mild weight may relieve a number of your signs of GERD. However, ensure to talk with a healthcare expert earlier than trying to shed pounds to deal with this circumstance.

8. Follow a low carb food plan

Growing proof shows that low carb diets may also relieve acid reflux disease disorder signs.

In fact, a few researchers suspect that undigested carbs may also motive bacterial overgrowth and elevated strain in the stomach, that could make contributions to acid reflux disease disorder.

Having too many undigested carbs on your digestive device regularly cannot simplest motive fueloline and bloating however additionally burping.

However, at the same time as a few research advise that low carb diets ought to enhance reflux signs, extra studies is wanted.

SUMMARY

Some studies shows that negative carb digestion and bacterial overgrowth in the small gut may also bring about acid reflux disease disorder. Low carb diets can be an powerful remedy, however in addition research are wished.

9. Limit your alcohol consumption

Drinking alcohol may also growth the severity of acid reflux disease disorder and heartburn.

In fact, a few research have proven that better alcohol consumption will be related to elevated signs of acid reflux disease disorder.

Alcohol aggravates signs with the aid of using growing belly acid, enjoyable the decrease esophageal sphincter, and impairing the capacity of the esophagus to clean out acid.

Although new studies is wanted, a few older research additionally display that consuming wine or beer will increase reflux signs, specially in comparison with consuming undeniable water.

SUMMARY

Excessive alcohol consumption can get worse acid reflux disease disorder signs. If you revel in heartburn, restricting your alcohol consumption may assist ease a number of your discomfort.

10. Don't drink an excessive amount of espresso

Studies have observed that espresso briefly relaxes the decrease esophageal sphincter, growing the chance of acid reflux disease disorder.

Some proof additionally factors towards caffeine as a probable motive. Similarly to espresso, caffeine relaxes the decrease esophageal sphincter, that could motive reflux.

Nevertheless, even though numerous research advise that espresso and caffeine may also get worse acid reflux disease disorder for a few humans, the proof isn't totally conclusive.

For example, one evaluation of observational research observed no widespread results of espresso consumption at the self-mentioned signs of GERD.

Yet, whilst researchers investigated the symptoms and symptoms of acid reflux disease disorder with a small camera, they observed espresso intake become related to extra acid harm in the esophagus .

Thus, whether or not espresso consumption worsens acid reflux disease disorder may also rely on the individual. If you locate espresso offers you heartburn, it's quality to virtually keep away from it or restrict your consumption.

SUMMARY

Evidence shows that espresso may also make acid reflux disease disorder and heartburn worse. If you experience like espresso worsens your signs, recall restricting your consumption.

CHAPTER FOUR

Limit your consumption
of carbonated drinks

Healthcare experts every so often endorse humans with GERD to restrict their consumption of carbonated drinks.

This is due to the fact research have located that normal intake of carbonated or fizzy drinks, together with tender drinks, membership soda, and seltzer, will be related to a better chance of reflux.

One take a look at observed that carbonated tender drinks, in particular, worsened sure acid reflux disease disorder signs, together with heartburn, fullness, and burping.

The predominant motive is that the carbon dioxide fueloline (the bubbles) in carbonated drinks reasons humans to burp extra regularly — an impact which can growth the quantity of acid escaping into the esophagus.

SUMMARY

Drinking carbonated drinks briefly will increase the frequency of burping, which may also sell acid reflux disease disorder. If they get worse your signs, attempt consuming much less or fending off them altogether.

12. Don't drink an excessive amount of citrus juice

Many forms of citrus juice, together with orange juice and grapefruit juice, are taken into consideration common triggers for heartburn.

These components are extraordinarily acidic and comprise compounds like ascorbic acid, that could motive indigestion in case you devour them in big quantities.

In addition to being acidic, sure compounds observed in citrus juice ought to worsen the liner of the esophagus.

While citrus juice likely doesn't motive acid reflux disease disorder directly, it may make your heartburn worse briefly.

SUMMARY

Some humans with acid reflux disease disorder document that consuming citrus juice makes their signs worse. Certain compounds in citrus juice, further to acids, also can worsen the liner of the esophagus.

13. Avoid mint, if wished

Peppermint and spearmint are common components used to make natural tea and upload taste to meals, candy, chewing gum, mouthwash, and toothpaste.

However, in addition they comprise sure compounds that would cause heartburn in a few humans.

For instance, a few research imply that peppermint oil ought to lower decrease esophageal sphincter strain, which may also motive heartburn.

Another take a look at confirmed that menthol, a compound observed in mint, ought to get worse reflux in humans with GERD.

Additionally, one older take a look at in humans with GERD confirmed that spearmint did now no longer have an effect on the decrease esophageal sphincter. Nevertheless, it observed that excessive doses of spearmint ought to get worse acid reflux disease disorder signs with the aid of using hectic the interior of the esophagus.

For this motive, it's quality to keep away from mint in case you experience that it makes your heartburn worse.

SUMMARY

A few research imply that mint and a number of the compounds it includes may also irritate heartburn and different reflux signs, however the proof is limited.

14. Limit excessive fats meals

Fried meals and a few different fatty meals will also be a cause for GERD. Some studies suggests they will cause heartburn. Examples include.

• fried meals

• potato chips

• pizza

• bacon

• sausage

High fats meals like those may also make contributions to heartburn with the aid of using inflicting bile salts to be launched into your digestive tract, which may also worsen your esophagus.

They additionally seem to stimulate the discharge of cholecystokinin (CCK), a hormone on your bloodstream that could loosen up the decrease esophageal sphincter, permitting belly contents again into the esophagus.

One take a look at checked out what came about whilst humans with GERD ate excessive fats meals. More than 1/2 of contributors who had mentioned meals triggers stated they skilled GERD signs after ingesting excessive fats, fried meals.

Moreover, as soon as those humans removed triggering meals from their food plan, the percentage of folks that skilled heartburn reduced from 93% to 44%.

More studies is wanted to find how excessive fats meals may cause GERD signs, together with heartburn, in addition to what styles of fat may have the most powerful results.

It's crucial to notice that fat are an crucial a part of a healthful food plan. Rather than fending off fat, purpose to devour them moderately from healthful sources, along with omega-three fatty acids from fatty fish and monounsaturated fat from olive oil or avocados.

SUMMARY

Foods which can be excessive in fats may also cause GERD signs, together with heartburn, in a few humans. However, extra studies is wanted.

The backside line

Heartburn is an uncomfortable difficulty that may be as a result of quite a few special factors.

Although there are numerous medicines and remedy alternatives to be had to ease heartburn, making some easy modifications in your food plan and life-style will also be beneficial.

Try a number of the hints above to locate what works a good way to lessen heartburn and acid reflux disease disorder.

THE END

www.ingramcontent.com/pod-product-compliance
Lightning Source LLC
Chambersburg PA
CBHW071003250726
48663CB00002B/363